CW00502464

The Easy Mediterranean Diet Cookbook

50 Flavourful Recipes Designed for an Healthy Eating

By Colleen Stevens

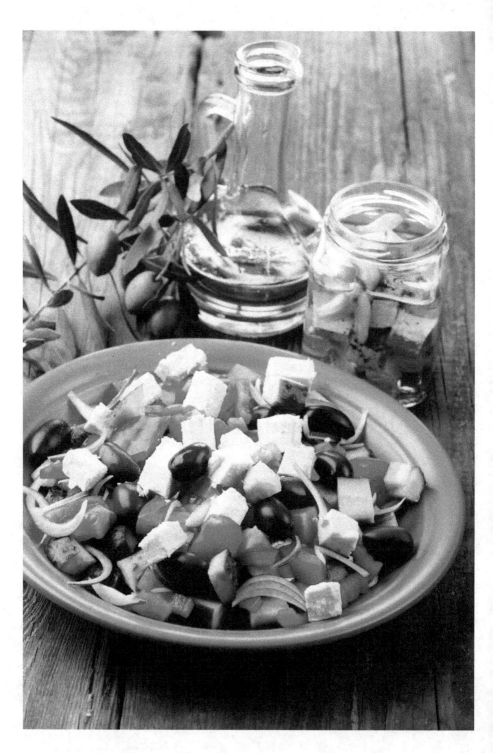

Table of Contents

3

Chapter 7: Dessert Recipes 98

Introduction

Mediterranean diet is based on the eating habits of the inhabitants of the regions along the Mediterranean Sea, mostly from Italy, Spain and Greece; it is considered more a life style then a diet, in fact it also promotes physical activity and proper liquid (mostly water) consumption.

Depending on fresh seasonal local foods there are no strict rules, because of the many cultural differences, but there are some common factors.

Mediterranean diet has become famous for its ability to reduce heart disease and obesity, thanks to the low consumption of unhealthy fats that increase blood glucose.

Mediterranean diet is mostly plant based, so it's rich of antioxidants; vegetables, fruits like apple and grapes, olive oil, whole grains, herbs, beans and nuts are consumed in large quantities.

Moderate amounts of poultry, eggs, dairy and seafood are also common aliments, accompanied by a little bit of red wine (some studies say that in small amount it helps to stay healthy).

Red meat and sweets like cookies and cakes are accepted but are more limited in quantity.

Foods to avoid:

- refined grains, such as white bread and pasta
- dough containing white flour refined oils (even canola oil and soybean oil)
- foods with added sugars (like pastries, sodas, and candies)
- processed meats processed or packaged foods

Chapter 1: Breakfast and Snack Recipes

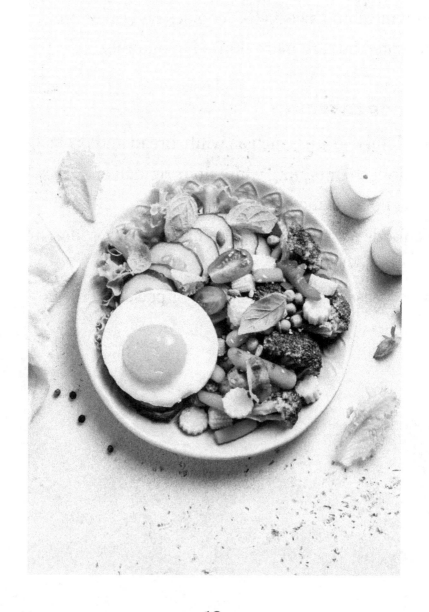

Chicken Souvlaki

Servings: 4 | Cooking: 2 min

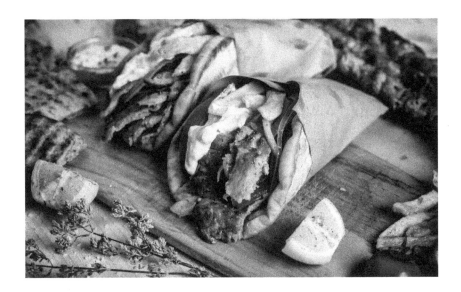

Ingredients

- 4 pieces (6-inch) pitas, cut into halves
- 2 cups roasted chicken breast skinless, boneless, and sliced
- 1/4 cup red onion, thinly sliced
- 1/2 teaspoon dried oregano
- 1/2 cup Greek yogurt, plain
- 1/2 cup plum tomato, chopped
- 1/2 cup cucumber, peeled, chopped
- 1/2 cup (2 ounces) feta cheese, crumbled

- 1 tablespoon olive oil, extra-virgin, divided
- 1 tablespoon fresh dill, chopped
- 1 cup iceberg lettuce, shredded
- 1 1/4 teaspoons minced garlic, bottled, divided

Directions

1. In a small mixing bowl, combine the yogurt, cheese, 1 teaspoon of the olive oil, and 1/4 teaspoon of the garlic until well mixed.
2. In a large skillet, heat the remaining olive oil over medium-high heat. Add the remaining 1 teaspoon garlic and the oregano; sauté for 20 seconds.
3. Add the chicken; cook for about 2 minutes or until the chicken are heated through.
4. Put 1/4 cup chicken into each pita halves. Top with 2 tablespoons yogurt mix, 2 tablespoons lettuce,1 tablespoon tomato, and 1 tablespoon cucumber. Divide the onion between the pita halves.

Nutrition:414 Cal, 13.7 g total fat (6.4 g sat. fat, 1.4 g poly. Fat, 4.7 g mono), 81 mg chol., 595 mg sodium, 38 g carb.,2 g fiber, 32.3 g protein.

Tahini Pine Nuts Toast

Servings: 2 | Cooking: 0 min

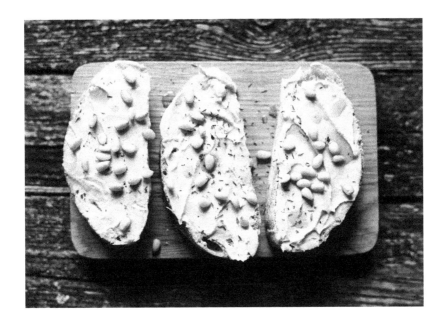

Ingredients

- 2 whole wheat bread slices, toasted
- 1 teaspoon water
- 1 tablespoon tahini paste
- 2 teaspoons feta cheese, crumbled
- Juice of ½ lemon
- 2 teaspoons pine nuts
- A pinch of black pepper

Directions

1. In a bowl, mix the tahini with the water and the lemon juice, whisk really well and spread over the toasted bread slices.
2. Top each serving with the remaining ingredients and serve for breakfast.

Nutrition: calories 142; fat 7.6; fiber 2.7; carbs 13.7; protein 5.8

Eggs and Veggies

Servings: 4 | Cooking: 15 min

Ingredients

- 2 tomatoes, chopped
- 2 eggs, beaten
- 1 bell pepper, chopped
- 1 teaspoon tomato paste
- ¼ cup of water
- 1 teaspoon butter
- ½ white onion, diced
- ½ teaspoon chili flakes
- 1/3 teaspoon sea salt

Directions

1. Put butter in the pan and melt it.
2. Add bell pepper and cook it for 3 minutes over the medium heat. Stir it from time to time.
3. After this, add diced onion and cook it for 2 minutes more.
4. Stir the vegetables and add tomatoes.

5. Cook them for 5 minutes over the medium-low heat.
6. Then add water and tomato paste. Stir well.
7. Add beaten eggs, chili flakes, and sea salt.
8. Stir well and cook menemen for 4 minutes over the medium-low heat.
9. The cooked meal should be half runny.

Nutrition: calories 67; fat 3.4; fiber 1.5; carbs 6.4; protein 3.8

Chili Scramble

Servings: 4 | Cooking: 15 min

Ingredients

- 3 tomatoes
- 4 eggs
- ¼ teaspoon of sea salt
- ½ chili pepper, chopped
- 1 tablespoon butter
- 1 cup water, for cooking

Directions

1. Pour water in the saucepan and bring it to boil.
2. Then remove water from the heat and add tomatoes.
3. Let the tomatoes stay in the hot water for 2-3 minutes.
4. After this, remove the tomatoes from water and peel them.
5. Place butter in the pan and melt it.
6. Add chopped chili pepper and fry it for 3 minutes over the medium heat.

7. Then chop the peeled tomatoes and add into the chili peppers.
8. Cook the vegetables for 5 minutes over the medium heat. Stir them from time to time.
9. After this, add sea salt and crack then eggs.
10. Stir (scramble) the eggs well with the help of the fork and cook them for 3 minutes over the medium heat.

Nutrition: calories 105; fat 7.4; fiber 1.1; carbs 4; protein 6.4

Pear Oatmeal

Servings: 4 | Cooking: 25 min

Ingredients

- 1 cup oatmeal
- 1/3 cup milk
- 1 pear, chopped
- 1 teaspoon vanilla extract
- 1 tablespoon Splenda
- 1 teaspoon butter
- ½ teaspoon ground cinnamon
- 1 egg, beaten

Directions

1. In the big bowl mix up together oatmeal, milk, egg, vanilla extract, Splenda, and ground cinnamon.
2. Melt butter and add it in the oatmeal mixture.
3. Then add chopped pear and stir it well.
4. Transfer the oatmeal mixture in the casserole mold and flatten gently. Cover it with the foil and secure edges.
5. Bake the oatmeal for 25 minutes at 350F.

Nutrition: calories 151; fat 3.9; fiber 3.3; carbs 23.6; protein 4.9

Mediterranean Frittata

Servings: 6 | Cooking: 15 min

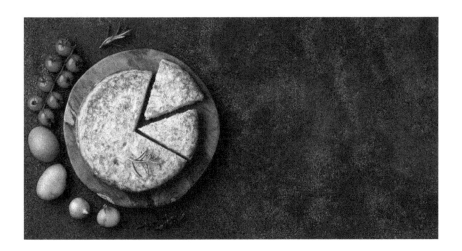

Ingredients

- 9 large eggs, lightly beaten
- 8 kalamata olives, pitted, chopped
- 1/4 cup olive oil
- 1/3 cup parmesan cheese, freshly grated
- 1/3 cup fresh basil, thinly sliced
- 1/2 teaspoon salt
- 1/2 teaspoon pepper
- 1/2 cup onion, chopped
- 1 sweet red pepper, diced
- 1 medium zucchini, cut to 1/2-inch cubes

- 1 package (4 ounce) feta cheese, crumbled

Directions

1. In a 10-inch oven-proof skillet, heat the olive oil until hot. Add the olives, zucchini, red pepper, and the onions, constantly stirring, until the vegetables are tender.
2. Ina bowl, mix the eggs, feta cheese, basil, salt, and pepper; pour in the skillet with vegetables. Adjust heat to medium-low, cover, and cook for about 10-12 minutes, or until the egg mixture is almost set.
3. Remove from the heat and sprinkle with the parmesan cheese. Transfer to the broiler.
4. With oven door partially open, broil 5 1/2 from the source of heat for about 2-3 minutes or until the top is golden. Cut into wedges.

Nutrition:288.5 Cal, 22.8 g total fat (7.8 g sat. fat), 301 mg chol., 656 mg sodium, 5.6 g carb.,1.2 g fiber,3.3g sugar, 15.2 g protein.

Mediterranean Egg Casserole

Servings: 8 | Cooking: 50 min

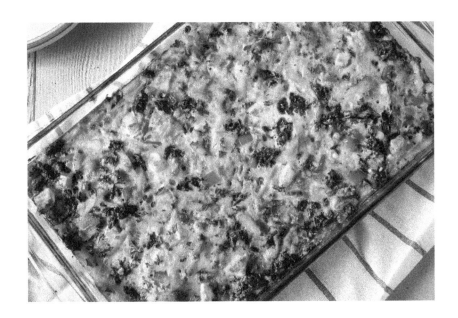

Ingredients

- 1 1/2 cups (6 ounces) feta cheese, crumbled
- 1 jar (6 ounces) marinated artichoke hearts, drained well, coarsely chopped
- 10 eggs
- 2 cups milk, low-fat
- 2 cups fresh baby spinach, packed, coarsely chopped
- 6 cups whole-wheat baguette, cut into 1-inch cubes

- 1 tablespoon garlic (about 4 cloves), finely chopped
- 1 tablespoon olive oil, extra-virgin
- 1/2 cup red bell pepper, chopped
- 1/2 cup Parmesan cheese, shredded
- 1/2 teaspoon pepper
- 1/2 teaspoon red pepper flakes
- 1/2 teaspoon salt
- 1/3 cup kalamata olives, pitted, halved
- 1/4 cup red onion, chopped
- 1/4 cup tomatoes (sun-dried) in oil, drained, chopped

Directions

1. Preheat oven to 350F.
2. Grease a 9x13-inch baking dish with olive oil cooking spray.
3. In an 8-inch non-stick pan over medium heat, heat the olive oil. Add the onions, garlic, and bell pepper; cook for about 3 minutes, frequently stirring, until slightly softened. Add the spinach; cook for about 1 minute or until starting to wilt.
4. Layer half of the baguette cubes in the prepared baking dish, then 1 cup of the eta, 1/4 cup

Parmesan, the bell pepper mix, artichokes, the olives, and the tomatoes. Top with the remaining baguette cubes and then with the remaining 1/2 cup of feta.

5. In a large mixing bowl, whisk the eggs and the low-fat milk together. Beat in the pepper, salt and the pepper. Pour the mix over the bread layer in the baking dish, slightly pressing down. Sprinkle with the remaining 1/4 cup Parmesan.

6. Bake for about 40-45 minutes, or until the center is set and the top is golden brown. Before serving, let stand for 15 minutes.

Nutrition:360 Cal, 21 g total fat (9 g sat. fat), 270 mg chol., 880 mg sodium, 24 g carb.,3 g fiber,7 g sugar, 20 g protein.

Milk Scones

Servings: 4 | Cooking: 10 min

Ingredients

- ½ cup wheat flour, whole grain
- 1 teaspoon baking powder
- 1 tablespoon butter, melted
- 1 teaspoon vanilla extract
- 1 egg, beaten
- ¾ teaspoon salt
- 3 tablespoons milk
- 1 teaspoon vanilla sugar

Directions

1. In the mixing bowl combine together wheat flour, baking powder, butter, vanilla extract, and egg. Add salt and knead the soft and non-sticky dough. Add more flour if needed.
2. Then make the log from the dough and cut it into the triangles.
3. Line the tray with baking paper.
4. Arrange the dough triangles on the baking paper and transfer in the preheat to the 360F oven.

5. Cook the scones for 10 minutes or until they are light brown.
6. After this, chill the scones and brush with milk and sprinkle with vanilla sugar.

Nutrition: calories 112; fat 4.4; fiber 0.5; carbs 14.3; protein 3.4

Herbed Eggs and Mushroom Mix

Servings: 4 | Cooking: 20 min

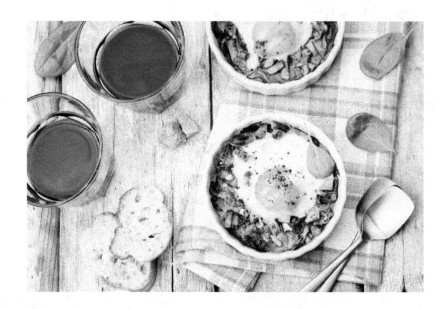

Ingredients

- 1 red onion, chopped
- 1 bell pepper, chopped
- 1 tablespoon tomato paste
- 1/3 cup water
- ½ teaspoon of sea salt
- 1 tablespoon butter
- 1 cup cremini mushrooms, chopped
- 1 tablespoon fresh parsley

- 1 tablespoon fresh dill
- 1 teaspoon dried thyme
- ½ teaspoon dried oregano
- ½ teaspoon paprika
- ½ teaspoon chili flakes
- ½ teaspoon garlic powder
- 4 eggs

Directions

1. Toss butter in the pan and melt it.
2. Then add chopped mushrooms and bell pepper.
3. Roast the vegetables for 5 minutes over the medium heat.
4. After this, add red onion and stir well.
5. Sprinkle the ingredients with garlic powder, chili flakes, dried oregano, and dried thyme. Mix up well
6. After this, add tomato paste and water.
7. Mix up the mixture until it is homogenous.
8. Then add fresh parsley and dill.
9. Cook the mixture for 5 minutes over the medium-high heat with the closed lid.

10. After this, stir the mixture with the help of the spatula well.

11. Crack the eggs over the mixture and close the lid.

12. Cook shakshuka for 10 minutes over the low heat.

Nutrition: calories 123; fat 7.5; fiber 1.7; carbs 7.8; protein 7.1

Leeks and Eggs Muffins

Servings: 2 | Cooking: 20 min

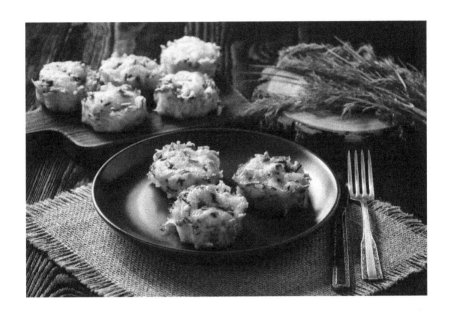

Ingredients

- 3 eggs, whisked
- ¼ cup baby spinach
- 2 tablespoons leeks, chopped
- 4 tablespoons parmesan, grated
- 2 tablespoons almond milk
- Cooking: spray
- 1 small red bell pepper, chopped
- Salt and black pepper to the taste

- 1 tomato, cubed
- 2 tablespoons cheddar cheese, grated

Directions

1. In a bowl, combine the eggs with the milk, salt, pepper and the rest of the ingredients except the cooking spray and whisk well.
2. Grease a muffin tin with the cooking spray and divide the eggs mixture in each muffin mould.
3. Bake at 380 degrees F for 20 minutes and serve them for breakfast.

Nutrition: calories 308; fat 19.4; fiber 1.7; carbs 8.7; protein 24.4

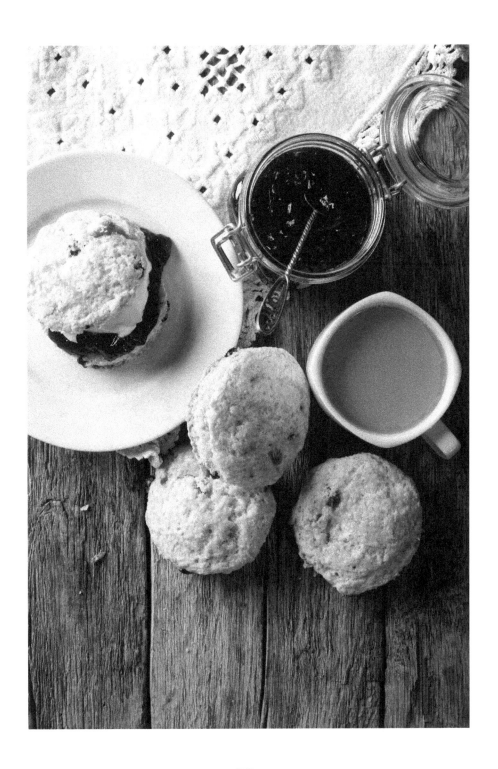

Chapter 2: Lunch & Dinner Recipes

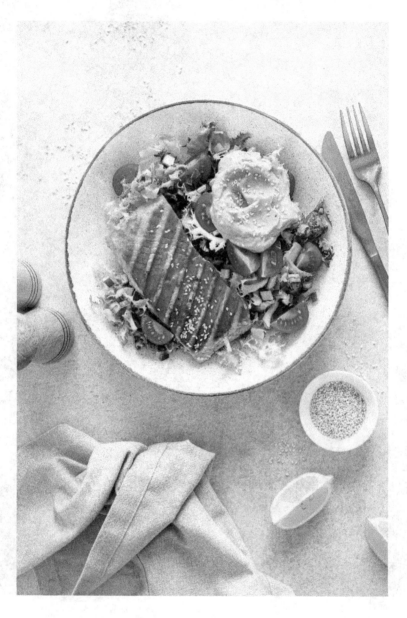

Slow-Cooked Pasta e Fagioli Soup

Servings: 6 | Kcal per serving: 457

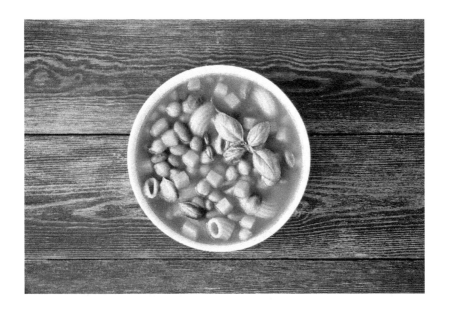

Ingredients

- 1/2 cup Parmigiano-Reggiano cheese (grated)
- 2 tablespoons extra-virgin olive oil
- 4 tablespoons chopped fresh basil (divided)
- 4 cups baby spinach
- 1 15-ounce can white beans with no-salt-added (rinsed)
- 1/4 teaspoon salt
- 4 teaspoons dried Italian seasoning

- 6 cups chicken broth (reduced-sodium)
- 4 cups whole-wheat rotini pasta (cooked)
- 1 pound cooked and diced chicken thighs (meal-prep sheet-pan)
- 1 cup celery (chopped)
- 1 cup carrots (chopped)
- 2 cups onion (minced)

Directions

1. Place celery, carrots, and onions in a Ziploc bag. In another Ziploc bag, put the cooked pasta along with the cooled cooked meat. Seal the bags and freeze. It will keep its freshness for up to 5 days.
2. Place the bags in the fridge the night before preparing this meal to defrost the ingredients.
3. Place the veggie mixture in a slow cooker. Add salt, Italian seasoning, and broth. Place the lid and cook for 7 hours on a low setting.
4. Add the pasta and meat, 2 tablespoons of basil, spinach, and beans. Cook for 45 more min.
5. Transfer to serving bowls. Add a bit of oil and top with basil and cheese.

Quinoa Bowl with Chickpeas

Servings: 4 | Kcal per serving: 479

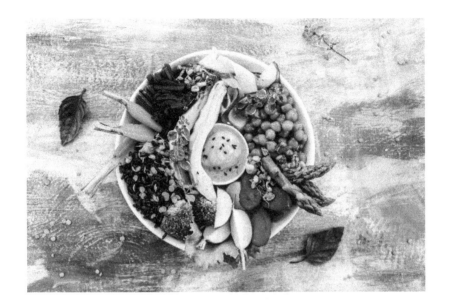

Ingredients

- 2 tablespoons fresh parsley (chopped)
- 1/4 cup feta cheese (crumbled)
- 1 cup cucumber (diced)
- 1 15-ounce can chickpeas (rinsed)
- 1/4 cup minced red onion
- 1/4 cup chopped Kalamata olives
- 2 cups cooked quinoa
- 1/4 teaspoon red pepper (crushed)

- 1/2 teaspoon ground cumin
- 1 teaspoon paprika
- 1 garlic clove (minced)
- 4 tablespoons extra-virgin olive oil (divided)
- 1/4 cup almonds (slivered)
- 1 7-ounce jar roasted red peppers (rinsed)

Directions

1. Puree red pepper, cumin, paprika, garlic, almonds, peppers, and 2 tablespoons of oil in a food processor.
2. Place the remaining oil in a bowl and add red onion, olives, and quinoa. Toss until combined.
3. Divide into bowls to serve. Top each with cucumber, chickpeas, and red pepper sauce. Sprinkle with parsley and cheese.

Salmon Served with Tomato and Fennel Couscous

Servings: 4 | Kcal per serving: 543

Ingredients

- 2 garlic cloves (sliced)
- 2 tablespoons pine nuts (toasted)
- 1/4 cup green olives (sliced)
- 1 1/2 cups chicken broth (low-sodium)
- 3 scallions (sliced)
- 1 cup whole-wheat Israeli couscous
- 2 fennel bulbs (sliced into wedges with a 1/2-inch thickness, reserve the fronds)
- 2 tablespoons extra-virgin olive oil (divided)
- 4 tablespoons sun-dried tomato pesto (divided)
- 1/4 teaspoon ground pepper
- 1/4 teaspoon salt
- 1 1/4 pounds salmon (skinned and quartered)
- 1 lemon (zest and slice into 8)

Directions

1. Rub salmon slices with salt and pepper. Spread them with 1 1/2 teaspoons pesto each.

2. Preheat a skillet over medium-high flame before adding oil. Cook half of the fennel for about 3 min or until the bottom gets browned. Transfer to a platter.

3. Turn heat to medium before adding the remaining oil. Cook the rest of the fennel and transfer to a platter.

4. Cook the scallions and couscous in the same skillet for a couple of min or until lightly toasted. Add 2 tablespoons of pesto, lemon zest, garlic, pine nuts, olives, and broth.

5. Place the fennel, salmon, and lemon slices on top of the couscous. Reduce heat and cover the skillet. Cook for 15 min or until the couscous is tender and the fish is done.

6. Add fennel fronds for garnishing when serving.

Edamame and Greens Salad with Avocado Slices

Servings: 1 | Kcal per serving: 405

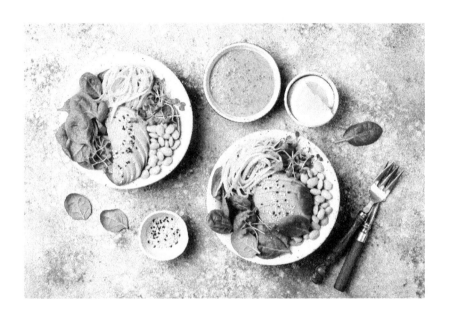

Ingredients

- 2 teaspoons extra-virgin olive oil
- 1 tablespoon fresh cilantro (chopped)
- Freshly ground pepper
- 1 tablespoon, plus 1 1/2 teaspoons red wine vinegar
- 1/2 cup peeled and shredded raw beet
- 1 cup edamame (shelled and thawed)

- 2 cups mixed salad greens
- 1/4 avocado (sliced)

Directions

1. Prepare the dressing. In a bowl, put oil, cilantro, and vinegar. Whisk until combined. Season with salt and pepper.
2. Place the beet, edamame, and salad greens on a plate. Drizzle with the dressing. Top with avocado slices, and serve.

Penne Pasta with Parsley Pesto

Servings: 2 | Kcal per serving: 630

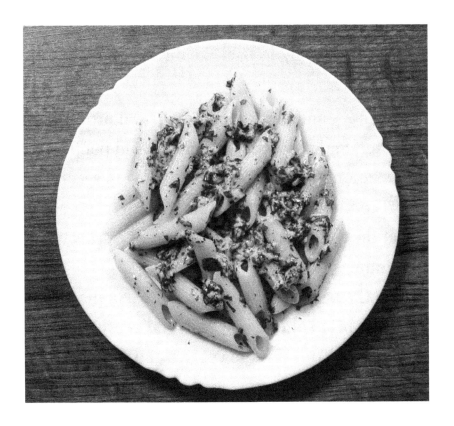

Ingredients

- 1 1/2 cups root veggies (roasted)
- 1/4 teaspoon ground black pepper
- 1/2 teaspoon kosher salt
- 2 tablespoons lemon juice
- 1 teaspoon lemon zest

- 1/3 cup extra-virgin olive oil
- 3 garlic cloves
- 4 cups lightly-packed parsley
- 4 ounces penne pasta (preferably chickpea penne, cooked according to package directions)

Directions

1. Put parsley and garlic cloves in a food processor or blender, and pulse until chopped. Add pepper, salt, lemon juice, and oil. Process for 15 seconds or until combined but still chunky.
2. Heat the roasted root veggies in the microwave for a minute.
3. Drain the pasta before transferring to a platter. Add the pesto and lemon zest, and gently toss until combined. Top with the veggies and serve.

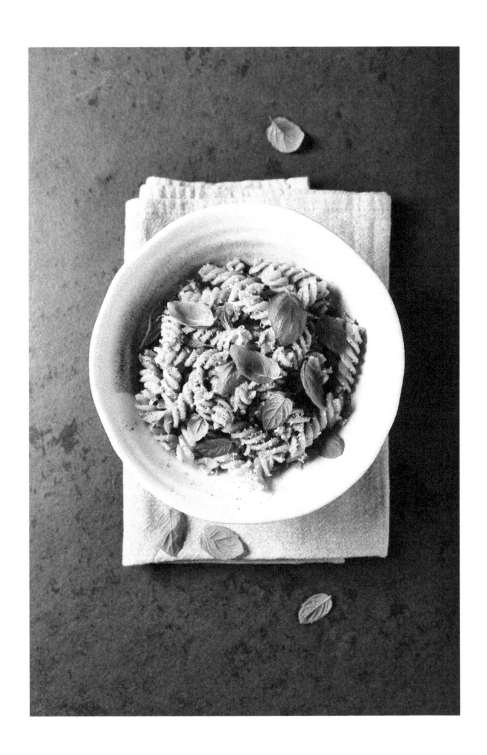

Chapter 3: Red Meat Recipes

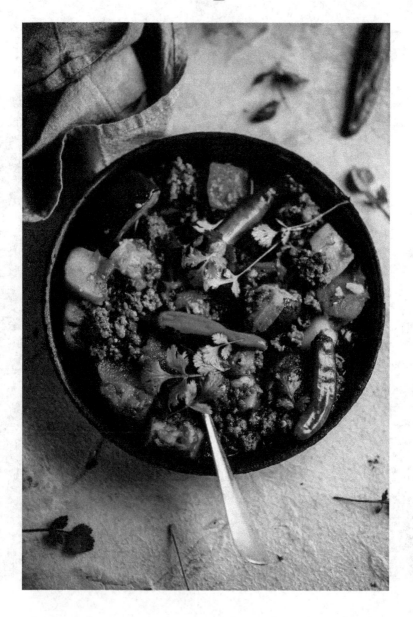

Hot Pork Meatballs

Servings: 2 | Cooking: 10 min

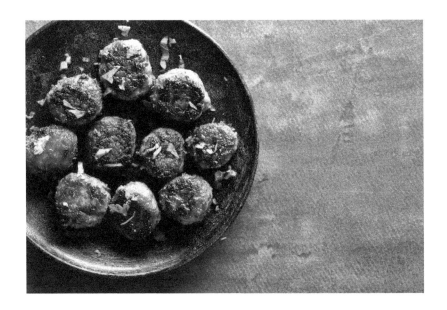

Ingredients

- 4 oz pork loin, grinded
- ½ teaspoon garlic powder
- ¼ teaspoon chili powder
- ¼ teaspoon cayenne pepper
- ¼ teaspoon ground black pepper
- ¼ teaspoon white pepper
- 1 tablespoon water
- 1 teaspoon olive oil

Directions

1. Mix up together grinded meat, garlic powder, cayenne pepper, ground black pepper, white pepper, and water.
2. With the help of the fingertips make the small meatballs.
3. Heat up olive oil in the skillet.
4. Arrange the kofte in the oil and cook them for 10 minutes totally. Flip the kofte on another side from time to time.

Nutrition: calories 162; fat 10.3; fiber 0.3; carbs 1; protein 15.7

Beef And Zucchini Skillet

Servings: 2 | Cooking: 20 min

Ingredients

- 2 oz ground beef
- ½ onion, sliced
- ½ bell pepper, sliced
- 1 tablespoon butter
- ½ teaspoon salt
- 1 tablespoon tomato sauce
- 1 small zucchini, chopped
- ½ teaspoon dried oregano

Directions

1. Place the ground beef in the skillet.
2. Add salt, butter, and dried oregano.
3. Mix up the meat mixture and cook it for 10 minutes.
4. After this, transfer the cooked ground beef in the bowl.
5. Place zucchini, bell pepper, and onion in the skillet (where the ground meat was cooking) and roast

the vegetables for 7 minutes over the medium heat or until they are tender.

6. Then add cooked ground beef and tomato sauce. Mix up well.
7. Cook the beef toss for 2-3 minutes over the medium heat.

Nutrition: calories 182; fat 8.7; fiber 0.1; carbs 0.3; protein 24.1

Greek Chicken Stew

Servings: 8 | Cooking: 1 Hour And 15minutes

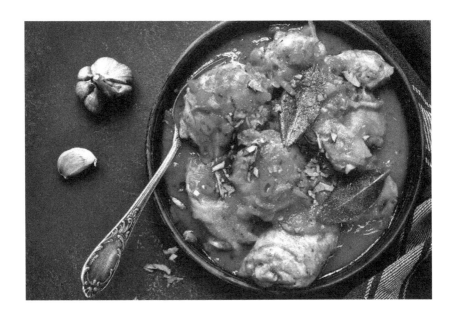

Ingredients

- 10 smalls shallots, peeled
- 1 cup olive oil
- 2 teaspoons butter
- 1 (4 pound) whole chicken, cut into pieces
- 2 cloves garlic, finely chopped
- ½ cup red wine
- 1 cup tomato sauce
- 2 tablespoons chopped fresh parsley

- salt and ground black pepper to taste
- 1 pinch dried oregano, or to taste
- 2 bay leaves
- 1 ½ cups chicken stock, or more if needed

Directions

1. In a large pot, fill half full of water and bring to a boil. Lightly salt the water and once boiling add shallots and boil uncovered for 3 minutes. Drain and quickly place on an ice bath for 5 minutes. Drain well.
2. In same pot, heat for 3 minutes and add oil and butter. Heat for 3 minutes.
3. Add chicken and shallots. Cook 15 minutes.
4. Add chopped garlic and cook for another 3 minutes or until garlic starts to turn golden.
5. Add red wine and tomato sauce. Deglaze pot.
6. Stir in bay leaves, oregano, pepper, salt, and parsley. Cook for 3 minutes.
7. Stir in chicken stock.
8. Cover and simmer for 40 minutes while occasionally stirring pot.
9. Serve and enjoy while hot with a side of rice if desired.

Nutrition: Calories: 574; Carbs: 6.8g; Protein: 31.8g; Fats: 45.3g

Meatloaf

Servings: 6 | Cooking: 35 min

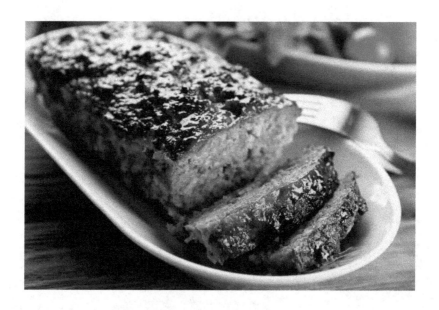

Ingredients

- 2 lbs ground beef
- 2 eggs, lightly beaten
- 1/4 tsp dried basil
- 3 tbsp olive oil
- 1/2 tsp dried sage
- 1 1/2 tsp dried parsley
- 1 tsp oregano
- 2 tsp thyme

- 1 tsp rosemary
- Pepper
- Salt

Directions

1. Pour 1 1/2 cups of water into the instant pot then place the trivet in the pot.
2. Spray loaf pan with cooking spray.
3. Add all ingredients into the mixing bowl and mix until well combined.
4. Transfer meat mixture into the prepared loaf pan and place loaf pan on top of the trivet in the pot.
5. Seal pot with lid and cook on high for 35 minutes.
6. Once done, allow to release pressure naturally for 10 minutes then release remaining using quick release. Remove lid.
7. Serve and enjoy.

Nutrition: Calories 365 Fat 18 g Carbohydrates 0.7 g Sugar 0.1 g Protein 47.8 g Cholesterol 190 mg

Tasty Lamb Ribs

Servings: 4 | Cooking: 2 Hours

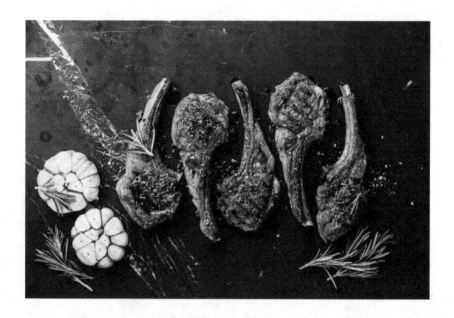

Ingredients

- 2 garlic cloves, minced
- ¼ cup shallot, chopped
- 2 tablespoons fish sauce
- ½ cup veggie stock
- 2 tablespoons olive oil
- 1 and ½ tablespoons lemon juice
- 1 tablespoon coriander seeds, ground
- 1 tablespoon ginger, grated

- Salt and black pepper to the taste
- 2 pounds lamb ribs

Directions

1. In a roasting pan, combine the lamb with the garlic, shallots and the rest of the ingredients, toss, introduce in the oven at 300 degrees F and cook for 2 hours.
2. Divide the lamb between plates and serve with a side salad.

Nutrition: calories 293; fat 9.1; fiber 9.6; carbs 16.7; protein 24.2

Chapter 4: Poultry Recipes

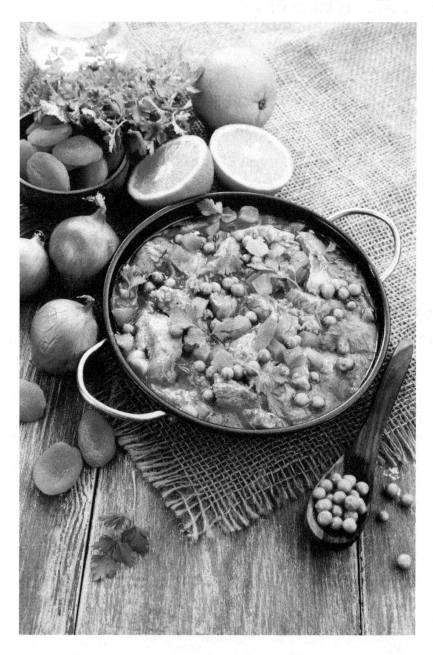

Chicken Skewers with Peanut Sauce

Preparation: 70 min | Cooking: 15 min | Servings: 2

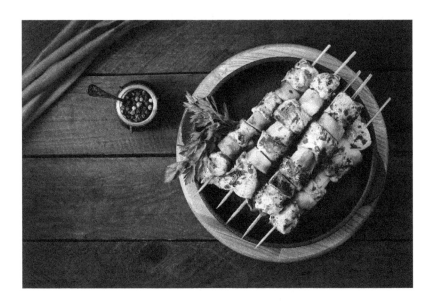

Ingredients

- 1-pound boneless skinless chicken breast, cut into chunks
- 3 tablespoons soy sauce (or coconut amino), divided
- ½ teaspoon plus ¼ teaspoon Sriracha sauce
- 3 teaspoons toasted sesame oil, divided
- 2 tablespoons peanut butter

Directions

1. In a large zip-top bag, mix chicken chunks with 2 tablespoons of soy sauce, ½ tsp. of Sriracha sauce and 2 tsp. of sesame oil. Cover and marinate for an h or so in the refrigerator or up to overnight.
2. If you are using wood 8-inch skewers, soak them in water for 30 min before using.
3. Preheat your grill pan or grill to low. Oil the grill pan with ghee.
4. Shred the chicken chunks onto the skewers.
5. Cook the skewers at low heat for 13 min, flipping halfway through.
6. Stir the peanut dipping sauce. Stir together the remaining 1 tablespoon of soy sauce, ¼ teaspoon of Sriracha sauce, 1 teaspoon of sesame oil, and the peanut butter. Season well.
7. Serve with peanut sauce.

Nutrition: 586 Calories: 29g Fat 75g Protein

Braised Chicken Thighs with Kalamata Olives

Preparation: 10 min | Cooking: 40 min | Servings: 4

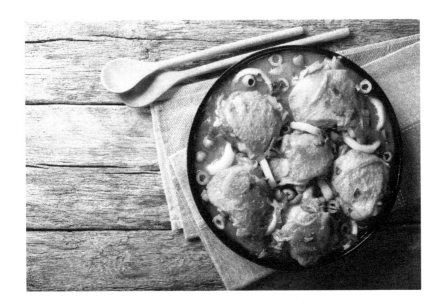

Ingredients

- 4 chicken thighs, skin on
- 2 tablespoons ghee
- ½ cup chicken broth
- lemon, ½ sliced and ½ juiced
- ½ cup pitted Kalamata olives

Directions

1. Preheat the oven to 375 degrees F.

2. Dry the chicken thighs using paper towels, and season with pink Himalayan salt and pepper.

3. In a medium oven-safe skillet or high-sided baking dish over medium-high heat, melt the ghee. When the ghee has melted and is hot, add the chicken thighs, skin-side down, and leave them for 8 min.

4. Cook the other side for 2 min. Around the chicken thighs, pour in the chicken broth, and add the lemon slices, lemon juice, and olives.

5. Bake for 30 min. Add the butter to the broth mixture.

6. Divide the chicken and olives between two plates and serve.

Nutrition: 567 Calories: 47g Fat 33g Protein:

Turkey And Salsa Verde

Servings: 4 | Cooking: 50 min

Ingredients

- 1 big turkey breast, skinless, boneless and cubed
- 1 and ½ cups Salsa Verde
- Salt and black pepper to the taste
- 1 tablespoon olive oil
- 1 and ½ cups feta cheese, crumbled
- ¼ cup cilantro, chopped

Directions

1. In a roasting pan greased with the oil combine the turkey with the salsa, salt and pepper and bake 400 degrees F for 50 minutes.
2. Add the cheese and the cilantro, toss gently, divide everything between plates and serve.

Nutrition: calories 332; fat 15.4; fiber 10.5; carbs 22.1; protein 34.5

Chili Chicken Fillets

Servings: 8 | Cooking: 7.5 Hours

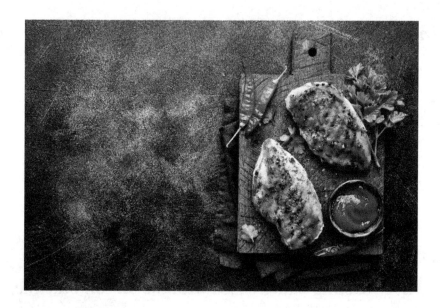

Ingredients

- 4 chicken fillets (5 oz each fillet)
- 8 bacon slices
- 1 teaspoon chili pepper
- 1 tablespoon olive oil
- ½ teaspoon salt
- 1 garlic clove, minced

Directions

1. Cut every chicken fillet lengthwise.

2. In the shallow bowl mix up together chili pepper, olive oil, minced garlic, and salt.
3. Rub every chicken fillet with oil mixture and wrap in the sliced bacon.
4. Transfer the prepared chicken fillets in the baking dish and cover with foil.
5. Bake the chicken fillets for 35 minutes at 365F.

Nutrition: calories 234; fat 15.2; fiber 0.5; carbs 8; protein 16.6

Chicken With Peas

Servings: 4 | Cooking: 30 min

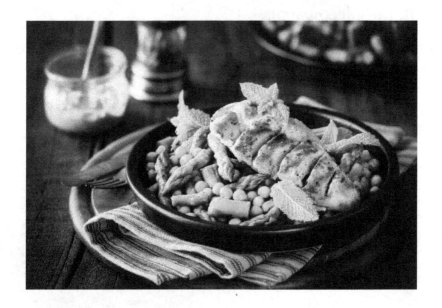

Ingredients

- 4 chicken fillets
- 1 teaspoon cayenne pepper
- 1 teaspoon salt
- 1 tablespoon mayonnaise
- 1 cup green peas
- ¼ cup of water
- 1 carrot, peeled, chopped

Directions

1. Sprinkle the chicken fillet with cayenne pepper and salt.
2. Line the baking tray with foil and place chicken fillets in it.
3. Then brush the chicken with mayonnaise.
4. Add carrot and green peas.
5. Then add water and cover the ingredients with foil.
6. Bake the chicken for 30 minutes at 355F.

Nutrition: calories 329 fat 12.3; fiber 2.3; carbs 7.9; protein 44.4

Chapter 5: Fish and Seafood Recipes

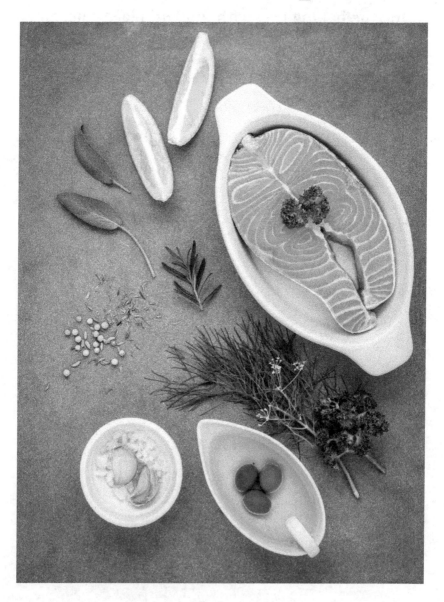

Honey Balsamic Salmon

Servings: 2 | Cooking: 3 min

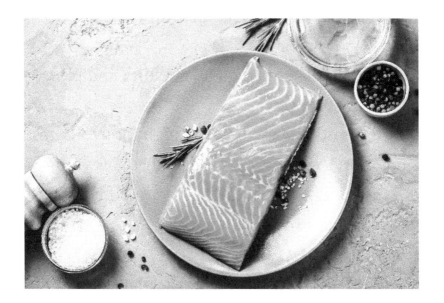

Ingredients

- 2 salmon fillets
- 1/4 tsp red pepper flakes
- 2 tbsp honey
- 2 tbsp balsamic vinegar
- 1 cup of water
- Pepper
- Salt

Directions

1. Pour water into the instant pot and place trivet in the pot.
2. In a small bowl, mix together honey, red pepper flakes, and vinegar.
3. Brush fish fillets with honey mixture and place on top of the trivet.
4. Seal pot with lid and cook on high for 3 minutes.
5. Once done, release pressure using quick release. Remove lid.
6. Serve and enjoy.

Nutrition: Calories 303 Fat 11 g Carbohydrates 17.6 g Sugar 17.3 g Protein 34.6 g Cholesterol 78 mg

Sage Salmon Fillet

Servings: 1 | Cooking: 25 min

Ingredients

- 4 oz salmon fillet
- ½ teaspoon salt
- 1 teaspoon sesame oil
- ½ teaspoon sage

Directions

1. Rub the fillet with salt and sage.
2. Place the fish in the tray and sprinkle it with sesame oil.
3. Cook the fish for 25 minutes at 365F.
4. Flip the fish carefully onto another side after 12 minutes of cooking.

Nutrition: calories 191; fat 11.6; fiber 0.1; carbs 0.2; protein 22

Seafood Stew Cioppino

Servings: 6 | Cooking: 40 min

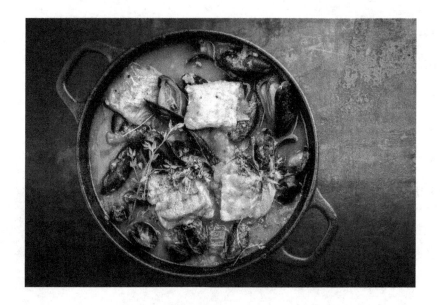

Ingredients

- ¼ cup Italian parsley, chopped
- ¼ tsp dried basil
- ¼ tsp dried thyme
- ½ cup dry white wine like pinot grigio
- ½ lb. King crab legs, cut at each joint
- ½ onion, chopped
- ½ tsp red pepper flakes (adjust to desired spiciness)

- 1 28-oz can crushed tomatoes
- 1 lb. mahi mahi, cut into ½-inch cubes
- 1 lb. raw shrimp
- 1 tbsp olive oil
- 2 bay leaves
- 2 cups clam juice
- 50 live clams, washed
- 6 cloves garlic, minced
- Pepper and salt to taste

Directions

1. On medium fire, place a stockpot and heat oil.
2. Add onion and for 4 minutes sauté until soft.
3. Add bay leaves, thyme, basil, red pepper flakes and garlic. Cook for a minute while stirring a bit.
4. Add clam juice and tomatoes. Once simmering, place fire to medium low and cook for 20 minutes uncovered.
5. Add white wine and clams. Cover and cook for 5 minutes or until clams have slightly opened.
6. Stir pot then add fish pieces, crab legs and shrimps. Do not stir soup to maintain the fish's shape. Cook while covered for 4 minutes or until

clams are fully opened; fish and shrimps are opaque and cooked.

7. Season with pepper and salt to taste.
8. Transfer Cioppino to serving bowls and garnish with parsley before serving.

Nutrition: Calories: 371; Carbs: 15.5 g; Protein: 62 g; Fat: 6.8 g

Shrimp and Lemon Sauce

Servings: 4 | Cooking: 15 min

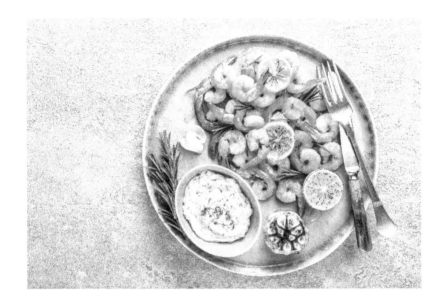

Ingredients

- 1 pound shrimp, peeled and deveined
- 1/3 cup lemon juice
- 4 egg yolks
- 2 tablespoons olive oil
- 1 cup chicken stock
- Salt and black pepper to the taste
- 1 cup black olives, pitted and halved
- 1 tablespoon thyme, chopped

Directions

1. In a bowl, mix the lemon juice with the egg yolks and whisk well.
2. Heat up a pan with the oil over medium heat, add the shrimp and cook for 2 minutes on each side and transfer to a plate.
3. Heat up a pan with the stock over medium heat, add some of this over the egg yolks and lemon juice mix and whisk well.
4. Add this over the rest of the stock, also add salt and pepper, whisk well and simmer for 2 minutes.
5. Add the shrimp and the rest of the ingredients, toss and serve right away.

Nutrition: calories 237; fat 15.3; fiber 4.6; carbs 15.4; protein 7.6

Feta Tomato Sea Bass

Servings: 4 | Cooking: 8 min

Ingredients

- 4 sea bass fillets
- 1 1/2 cups water
- 1 tbsp olive oil
- 1 tsp garlic, minced
- 1 tsp basil, chopped
- 1 tsp parsley, chopped
- 1/2 cup feta cheese, crumbled
- 1 cup can tomatoes, diced
- Pepper
- Salt

Directions

1. Season fish fillets with pepper and salt.
2. Pour 2 cups of water into the instant pot then place steamer rack in the pot.
3. Place fish fillets on steamer rack in the pot.
4. Seal pot with lid and cook on high for 5 minutes.
5. Once done, release pressure using quick release. Remove lid.

6. Remove fish fillets from the pot and clean the pot.
7. Add oil into the inner pot of instant pot and set the pot on sauté mode.
8. Add garlic and sauté for 1 minute.
9. Add tomatoes, parsley, and basil and stir well and cook for 1 minute.
10. Add fish fillets and top with crumbled cheese and cook for a minute.
11. Serve and enjoy.

Nutrition: Calories 219 Fat 10.1 g Carbohydrates 4 g Sugar 2.8 g Protein 27.1 g Cholesterol 70 mg

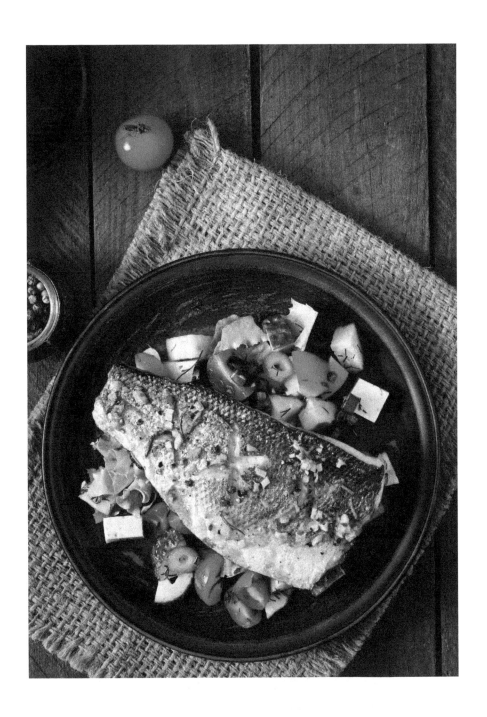

Chapter 6: Salads & Side Dishes

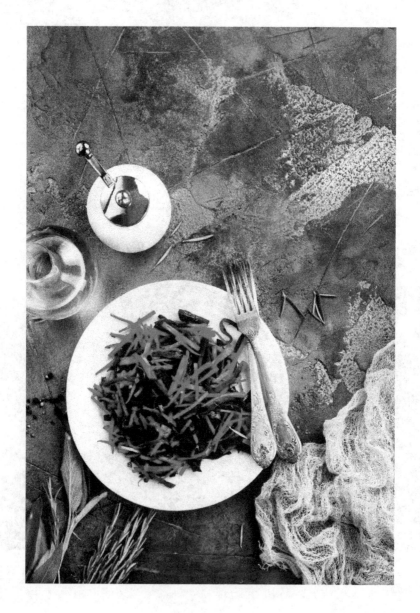

Okra and Tomato Casserole

Preparation: 25 min | Cooking: 26 min | Servings: 4

Ingredients

- 3 lb. okra, trimmed
- 3tomatoes, cut into wedges
- 2 garlic cloves, chopped
- 1 cup fresh parsley leaves, finely cut
- 1 tbsp. extra virgin olive oil

Directions

1. In a deep ovenproof baking dish, combine okra, sliced tomatoes, olive oil and garlic.
2. Toss to combine and bake in a preheated to 350 degrees F oven for 45 min. Drizzle with parsley and serve.

Nutrition: 304 calories; 48g fat; 13g protein

Spicy Baked Feta with Tomatoes

Preparation: 15 min | Cooking: 22 min | Servings: 4

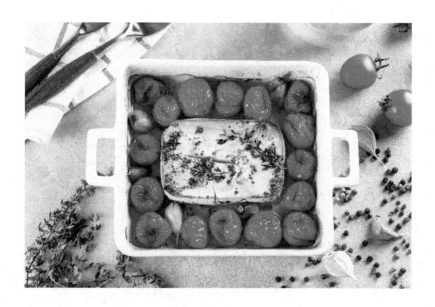

Ingredients

- 2 lb. feta cheese, cut in slices
- ripe tomatoes, sliced
- 1 onion, sliced
- 1 tbsp. extra virgin olive oil
- 1/2 tbsp. hot paprika

Directions

1. Preheat the oven to 430F

2. In an ovenproof baking dish, arrange the slices of onions and tomatoes overlapping slightly but not too much. Sprinkle with olive oil.
3. Bake for 5 min then place the feta slices on top of the vegetables. Sprinkle with hot paprika. Bake for 15 more min and serve.

Nutrition: 303 calories; 46g fat; 12g protein

Cream Of Artichoke Soup

Servings: 6 | Cooking: 45 min

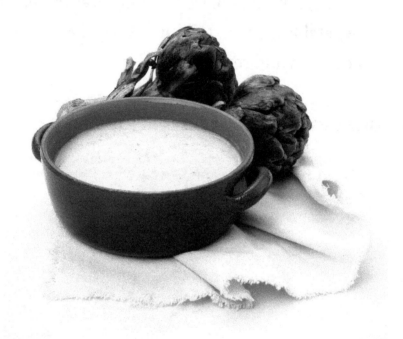

Ingredients

- 2 tablespoons olive oil
- 2 shallots, chopped
- 2 garlic cloves, chopped
- 1 jar artichoke hearts, chopped
- 2 pears, peeled and cubed
- 2 cups vegetable stock

- 1 cup water
- Salt and pepper to taste
- ¼ cup heavy cream

Directions

1. Heat the oil in a soup pot and stir in the shallots and garlic. Cook for 2 minutes until softened.
2. Add the artichoke hearts, pears, stock and water, as well as salt and pepper.
3. Cook for 15 minutes then remove from heat and stir in the cream.
4. Puree the soup with an immersion blender and serve the soup fresh.

Nutrition: Calories:116 Fat:6.7g Protein:1.5g Carbohydrates:14.8g

Tuscan Cabbage Soup

Servings: 8 | Cooking: 1 Hour

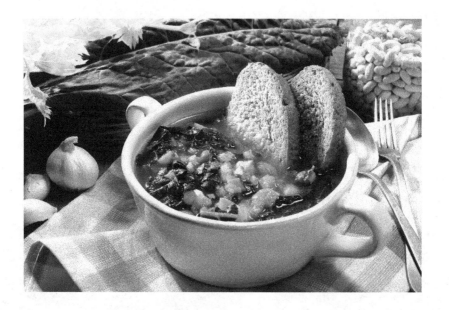

Ingredients

- 2 tablespoons olive oil
- 2 sweet onions, chopped
- 2 carrots, grated
- 1 celery stalk, chopped
- 1 can diced tomatoes
- 1 cabbage, shredded
- 2 cups vegetable stock
- 2 cups water

- 1 lemon, juiced
- 1 thyme sprig
- 1 oregano sprig
- 1 basil sprig
- Salt and pepper to taste

Directions

1. Heat the oil in a soup pot and stir in the onions, carrots and celery.
2. Cook for 5 minutes then stir in the rest of the ingredients.
3. Season with salt and pepper to taste and cook on low heat for 25 minutes.
4. Serve the soup warm.

Nutrition: Calories:58 Fat:3.6g Protein:1.0g Carbohydrates:6.6g

Smoky Sausage Soup

Servings: 8 | Cooking: 45 min

Ingredients

- 2 tablespoons olive oil
- 2 smoked chicken sausages, sliced
- 2 fresh chicken sausages, sliced
- 2 carrots, sliced
- 1 sweet onion, chopped
- 1 celery stalk, sliced
- 1 can diced tomatoes
- ½ cup short pasta
- 2 cups vegetable stock
- 4 cups water
- Salt and pepper to taste
- 2 tablespoons chopped parsley
- 2 tablespoons chopped cilantro

Directions

1. Heat the oil in a soup pot and stir in the sausages. Cook for 5 minutes then add the carrots, sweet onion, celery and tomatoes and continue cooking for another 5 minutes.

2. Add the stock, pasta, water, salt and pepper and cook for 20 minutes.
3. When done, stir in the parsley and cilantro and serve the soup warm and fresh.

Nutrition: Calories:48 Fat:3.6g Protein:0.6g Carbohydrates:4.0g

Grilled Salmon Summer Salad

Servings: 4 | Cooking: 30 min

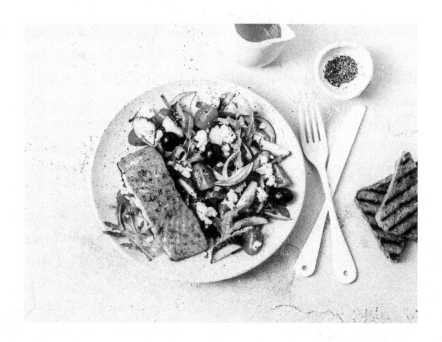

Ingredients

- Salmon fillets - 2
- Salt and pepper - to taste
- Vegetable stock - 2 cups
- Bulgur - 1 2 cup
- Cherry tomatoes - 1 cup, halved
- Sweet corn - 1 2 cup
- Lemon - 1, juiced

- Green olives - 1 2 cup, sliced
- Cucumber - 1, cubed
- Green onion - 1, chopped
- Red pepper - 1, chopped
- Red bell pepper - 1, cored and diced

Directions

1. Heat a grill pan on medium and then place salmon on, seasoning with salt and pepper. Grill both sides of salmon until brown and set aside.
2. Heat stock in sauce pan until hot and then add in bulgur and cook until liquid is completely soaked into bulgur.
3. Mix salmon, bulgur and all other Ingredients in a salad bowl and again add salt and pepper, if desired, to suit your taste.
4. Serve salad as soon as completed.

Dill Beets Salad

Servings: 6 | Cooking: 0 min

Ingredients

- 2 pounds beets, cooked, peeled and cubed
- 2 tablespoons olive oil
- 1 tablespoon lemon juice
- 2 tablespoons balsamic vinegar
- 1 cup feta cheese, crumbled
- 3 small garlic cloves, minced
- 4 green onions, chopped
- 5 tablespoons parsley, chopped
- Salt and black pepper to the taste

Directions

1. In a bowl, mix the beets with the oil, lemon juice and the rest of the ingredients, toss and serve as a side dish.

Nutrition: calories 268; fat 15.5; fiber 5.1; carbs 25.7; protein 9.6

Green Couscous With Broad Beans, Pistachio, And Dill

Servings: 4 | Cooking: 8 min

Ingredients

- 200 g fresh or frozen broad beans, podded
- 2 teaspoons ground ginger
- 2 tablespoons spring onion, thinly sliced
- 2 tablespoons pistachio kernels, roughly chopped
- 2 tablespoons lemon juice, and wedges to serve
- Dill, chopped - 1/4 cup
- Olive oil, extra-virgin - 1/4 cup (about 60 ml)
- 1/2 onion, thinly sliced
- Watercress, leaves picked - 1/2 bunch
- 1/2 avocado, chopped
- 1 green bell pepper, thinly sliced
- 1 garlic clove, crushed
- 1 cup (about 200 g) whole-grain couscous
- 1 1/2 cups boiling water

Directions

1. In a heat-safe bowl, toss the couscous with the ginger and the onion. Stir in the boiling water, cover and let stand for 5 minutes.

2. Meanwhile, cook the beans for about 3 minutes in boiling salted water, drain, and refresh under running cold water; discard the outer skins.

3. With a fork, fluff the couscous. Add the beans, avocado, bell pepper, spring onion, and dill.

4. In a bowl, whisk the olive oil, lemon juice, and garlic; toss with the couscous. Scatter the pistachio over the mix, serve with cress and the lemon wedges.

Nutrition: 608 cal, 25.40 g total fat (4 g sat. fat), 51.50 g carb, 18.10 g protein, 45 mg sodium, and 11 g fiber.

Bell Peppers Salad

Servings: 6 | Cooking: 0 min

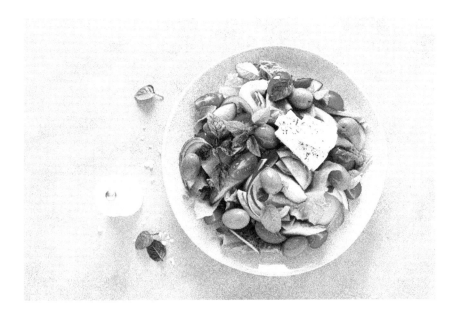

Ingredients

- 2 green bell peppers, cut into thick strips
- 2 red bell peppers, cut into thick strips
- 2 tablespoons olive oil
- 1 garlic clove, minced
- ½ cup goat cheese, crumbled
- A pinch of salt and black pepper

Directions

1. In a bowl, mix the bell peppers with the garlic and the other ingredients, toss and serve.

Nutrition: calories 193; fat 4.5; fiber 2; carbs 4.3; protein 3

Thyme Corn And Cheese Mix

Servings: 4 | Cooking: 0 min

Ingredients

- 1 tablespoon olive oil
- 1 teaspoon thyme, chopped
- 1 cup scallions, sliced
- 2 cups corn
- Salt and black pepper to the taste
- 2 tablespoons blue cheese, crumbled
- 1 tablespoon chives, chopped

Directions

1. In a salad bowl, combine the corn with scallions, thyme and the rest of the ingredients, toss, divide between plates and serve.

Nutrition: calories 183; fat 5.5; fiber 7.5; carbs 14.5

Chapter 7: Dessert Recipes

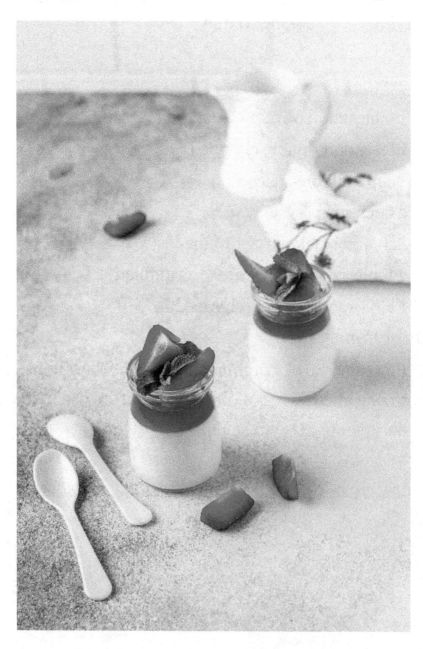

Creamy Pie

Servings: 6 | Cooking: 30 min

Ingredients

- ¼ cup lemon juice
- 1 cup cream
- 4 egg yolks
- 4 tablespoons Erythritol
- 1 tablespoon cornstarch
- 1 teaspoon vanilla extract
- 3 tablespoons butter
- 6 oz wheat flour, whole grain

Directions

1. Mix up together wheat flour and butter and knead the soft dough.
2. Put the dough in the round cake mold and flatten it in the shape of pie crust.
3. Bake it for 15 minutes at 365F.
4. Meanwhile, make the lemon filling: Mix up together cream, egg yolks, and lemon juice. When the liquid is smooth, start to heat it up over the medium heat. Stir it constantly.

5. When the liquid is hot, add vanilla extract, cornstarch, and Erythritol. Whisk well until smooth.
6. Brin the lemon filling to boil and remove it from the heat.
7. Cool it to the room temperature.
8. Cook the pie crust to the room temperature.
9. Pour the lemon filling over the pie crust, flatten it well and leave to cool in the fridge for 25 minutes.

Nutrition: calories 225; fat 11.4; fiber 0.8; carbs 34.8; protein 5.2

Hazelnut Pudding

Servings: 8 | Cooking: 40 min

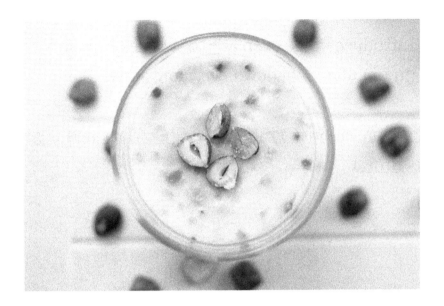

Ingredients

- 2 and ¼ cups almond flour
- 3 tablespoons hazelnuts, chopped
- 5 eggs, whisked
- 1 cup stevia
- 1 and 1/3 cups Greek yogurt
- 1 teaspoon baking powder
- 1 teaspoon vanilla extract

Directions

1. In a bowl, combine the flour with the hazelnuts and the other ingredients, whisk well, and pour into a cake pan lined with parchment paper,
2. Introduce in the oven at 350 degrees F, bake for 30 minutes, cool down, slice and serve.

Nutrition: calories 178; fat 8.4; fiber 8.2; carbs 11.5; protein 1.4

Mediterranean Cheesecakes

Servings: 1 Cheesecake | Cooking: 20 min

Ingredients

- 4 cups shredded phyllo (kataifi dough)
- 1/2 cup butter, melted
- 12 oz. cream cheese
- 1 cup Greek yogurt
- 3/4 cup confectioners' sugar
- 1 TB. vanilla extract
- 2 TB. orange blossom water
- 1 TB. orange zest
- 2 large eggs
- 1 cup coconut flakes

Directions

1. Preheat the oven to 450°F.
2. In a large bowl, and using your hands, combine shredded phyllo and melted butter, working the two together and breaking up phyllo shreds as you work.
3. Using a 12-cup muffin tin, add 1/3 cup shredded phyllo mixture to each tin, and press down to form

crust on the bottom of the cup. Bake crusts for 8 minutes, remove from the oven, and set aside.

4. In a large bowl, and using an electric mixer on low speed, blend cream cheese and Greek yogurt for 1 minute.

5. Add confectioners' sugar, vanilla extract, orange blossom water, and orange zest, and blend 1 minute.

6. Add eggs, and blend for about 30 seconds or just until eggs are incorporated.

7. Lightly coat the sides of each muffin tin with cooking spray.

8. Pour about 1/3 cup cream cheese mixture over crust in each tin. Do not overflow.

9. Bake for 12 minutes.

10. Spread shredded coconut on a baking sheet, and place in the oven with cheesecakes to toast for 4 or 5 minutes or until golden brown. Remove from the oven, and set aside.

11. Remove cheesecakes from the oven, and cool for 1 hour on the countertop.

12. Place the tin in the refrigerator, and cool for 1 more hour.

13. To serve, dip a sharp knife in warm water and then run it along the sides of cheesecakes to loosen from the tin. Gently remove cheesecakes and place on a serving plate.
14. Sprinkle with toasted coconut flakes, and serve.

Melon Cucumber Smoothie

Servings: 2 | Cooking: 5 min

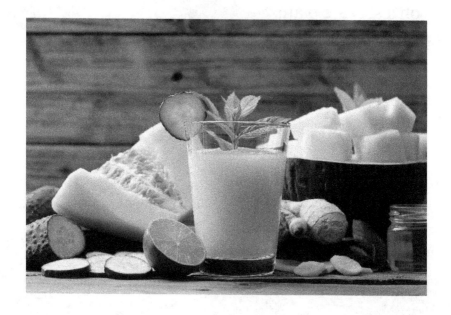

Ingredients

- ½ cucumber
- 2 slices of melon
- 2 tablespoons lemon juice
- 1 pear, peeled and sliced
- 3 fresh mint leaves
- ½ cup almond milk

Directions

1. Place all Ingredients: in a blender.

2. Blend until smooth.

3. Pour in a glass container and allow to chill in the fridge for at least 30 minutes.

Nutrition: Calories per serving: 253; Carbs: 59.3g; Protein: 5.7g; Fat: 2.1g

Mediterranean Style Fruit Medley

Servings: 7 | Cooking: 5 min

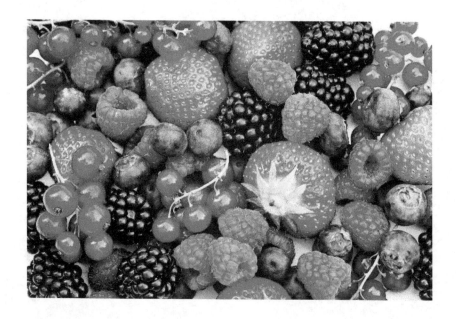

Ingredients

- 4 fuyu persimmons, sliced into wedges
- 1 ½ cups grapes, halved
- 8 mint leaves, chopped
- 1 tablespoon lemon juice
- 1 tablespoon honey
- ½ cups almond, toasted and chopped

Directions

1. Combine all Ingredients: in a bowl.
2. Toss then chill before serving.

Nutrition: Calories per serving:159; Carbs: 32g; Protein: 3g; Fat: 4g

CPSIA information can be obtained
at www.ICGtesting.com
Printed in the USA
BVHW092054080621
609008BV00003B/511

9 781911 688853